THE HIDDEN STRUGGLE

Common Causes of Infertility in Both Sexes

By

Martha T. Nye

TABLE OF CONTENTS

INTRODUCTION

The main characteristic of infertility, a complicated and diverse condition that affects both males and females, is the inability to become pregnant after one year of regular, unprotected sex. In women, ovulatory disorders, which hinder the release of mature eggs from the ovaries, are among the leading causes. One major cause is polycystic ovarian syndrome (PCOS), which leads to hormonal imbalances that interfere with ovulation. Other issues include endometriosis: a disorder whereby tissue similar to the uterus lining grows outside it causing inflammation and scarring that may obstruct reproductive organs, as well as ovarian reserve declination due to age, resulting in lower number and quality of eggs.

In men, infertility is often linked to sperm production or function problems. Low sperm count, poor motility or abnormal sperm morphology can all prevent fertilization from occurring for instance. Hormonal imbalances too play significant roles along with diseases affecting reproduction systems and hereditary defects such as Klinefelter syndrome. Moreover, unhealthy lifestyle choices like tobacco smoking, having too much alcohol within a short time period, obesity and exposure to environmental toxins also negatively influence sperm health.

In men and women, infertility may also arise due to structural problems. The egg cannot be reached by sperm of the women who have blocked fallopian tubes that are usually caused by pelvic inflammatory disease (PID) or surgery done before. Variable factors such as congenital malformations in the systems responsible for carrying sperms and illnesses like varicoceles can result in blockages in the sperm delivery system of males.

CHAPTER 1: HORMONAL IMBALANCES

Hormonal imbalances are a leading cause of infertility in both men and women. Several key hormones play critical roles in regulating fertility and reproduction, and imbalances in these hormones can significantly impact one's ability to conceive.

Impact of Hormonal Imbalances on Female Fertility

- Estrogen Imbalance

Estrogen imbalance can disrupt the menstrual cycle, making it difficult to track ovulation and the fertile window. High or low estrogen levels can also contribute to conditions like endometriosis, polycystic ovarian syndrome (PCOS), and uterine fibroids, all of which can impair fertility.

- Progesterone Imbalance

Progesterone imbalance, with low levels in particular, can lead to irregular periods and difficulty conceiving. Progesterone is essential for preparing the uterine lining for implantation and supporting early pregnancy.

- Follicle-Stimulating Hormone (FSH) and Luteinizing Hormone (LH) Imbalance

Follicle-stimulating hormone (FSH) and luteinizing hormone (LH) play key roles in regulating the menstrual cycle and ovulation. Imbalances in these hormones can disrupt ovulation, causing ovulatory dysfunction and infertility.

- Thyroid Hormone Imbalance

Thyroid hormone imbalances, both hypothyroidism and hyperthyroidism, can also impact fertility by affecting ovulation, menstrual cycles, and other reproductive functions.

- Other Hormone Imbalances

Other hormones like anti-Müllerian hormone (AMH), prolactin, and testosterone can also contribute to fertility issues when out of balance.

Impact of Hormonal Imbalances on Male Fertility

In men, hormonal imbalances like low testosterone can impair sperm production and quality, leading to male factor infertility.

- Testosterone Imbalance:

Low testosterone levels (hypogonadism) can impair sperm production, reduce sex drive, and lead to erectile dysfunction - all of which can contribute to male infertility. Excessive estrogen levels in men can also reduce sperm concentration and motility

- Follicle-Stimulating Hormone (FSH) and Luteinizing Hormone (LH) Imbalance:

FSH and LH play crucial roles in regulating sperm production. Imbalances in these hormones can disrupt spermatogenesis and lead to low sperm count, poor sperm quality, and infertility.

- Prolactin Imbalance:

High prolactin levels (hyperprolactinemia) can inhibit the production of gonadotropin-releasing hormone, leading to decreased FSH, LH, and testosterone - ultimately impacting sperm production.

- Thyroid Hormone Imbalance:

Both hypothyroidism and hyperthyroidism can affect male fertility by disrupting the hormonal balance and impacting sexual function, sperm production, and overall reproductive health.

Conditions Associated with Hormonal Imbalances and Infertility

- Polycystic Ovarian Syndrome (PCOS)

PCOS is a condition characterized by the production of higher-than-normal levels of androgens (male hormones) in the female body. PCOS can cause cysts to develop on the ovaries, irregular menstrual cycles, and can lead to fertility problems.

- Thyroid Disorders

Both an overactive thyroid (hyperthyroidism) and an underactive thyroid (hypothyroidism) can cause hormonal imbalances that affect fertility. Thyroid disorders can disrupt the menstrual cycle and ovulation, making it difficult to conceive.

- Hyperprolactinemia

Hyperprolactinemia is a condition characterized by elevated levels of the hormone prolactin. High prolactin levels can interfere with the production of other hormones necessary for ovulation and fertility.

Diagnosing Hormonal Imbalances

Identifying and addressing the underlying hormonal imbalance is crucial for restoring fertility. Treatment may involve medications to regulate hormone levels, lifestyle changes, or in some cases, surgery. Working closely with a fertility specialist is important for navigating hormonal imbalances and finding the right treatment approach.

Treatment Options for Hormonal Imbalances and Infertility

- Medications

Medications can be used to regulate hormone levels and address specific imbalances. For example, clomiphene citrate or letrozole may be prescribed to stimulate ovulation in women with ovulatory dysfunction, while metformin can help manage PCOS.

- Lifestyle Changes

Lifestyle changes, such as maintaining a healthy weight, exercising regularly, and managing stress, can also help improve hormonal balance and fertility. Dietary modifications, such as reducing processed foods and increasing nutrient-dense whole foods, may also be beneficial.

- Assisted Reproductive Technology (ART)

In some cases, assisted reproductive technology (ART) may be necessary to overcome infertility caused by hormonal imbalances. ART procedures, such as in vitro fertilization (IVF), can help bypass certain fertility issues and increase the chances of conception.

Preventing Hormonal Imbalances

While some hormonal imbalances are unavoidable due to underlying medical conditions, there are steps one can take to maintain hormonal balance and support fertility:

- Maintaining a healthy weight.

- Engaging in regular physical activity.
- Managing stress through relaxation techniques and mindfulness practices.
- Avoiding exposure to endocrine-disrupting chemicals found in certain plastics, personal care products, and pesticides.
- Quitting smoking and limiting alcohol consumption.
- Ensuring adequate sleep and rest.

Hormonal imbalances are a significant contributor to infertility in both men and women. Imbalances in estrogen, progesterone, FSH, LH, thyroid hormones, and other key reproductive hormones can disrupt ovulation, menstrual cycles, and other critical fertility processes. Proper diagnosis and targeted treatment of these hormonal imbalances, through medications, lifestyle changes, or ART, are essential for improving the chances of conception.

CHAPTER 2: GENETIC FACTORS

Genetic factors play a significant role in determining fertility in both men and women. Several genetic disorders and chromosomal abnormalities can contribute to infertility, impacting various aspects of the reproductive system.

Genetic Factors Affecting Female Fertility
- Turner Syndrome

Turner syndrome is a chromosomal disorder that affects females, characterized by the partial or complete absence of one of the X chromosomes. This condition can lead to ovarian dysfunction, resulting in primary ovarian insufficiency (POI) and infertility.

- Fragile X Premutation

The fragile X premutation is a genetic change in the FMR1 gene located on the X chromosome. This change can cause the ovaries to be less productive, limiting fertility and potentially leading to POI.

- Polycystic Ovarian Syndrome (PCOS)

PCOS is a hormonal disorder that affects women of reproductive age. While the exact cause is not fully understood, genetic factors play a significant role in the development of PCOS. Studies have identified several genes associated with PCOS, including DENND1A, LHCGR, and FSHR.

Genetic Factors Affecting Male Fertility
- Klinefelter Syndrome

Klinefelter syndrome is a chromosomal disorder in males characterized by the presence of an additional X chromosome (47, XXY). This condition can lead to small testes, reduced testosterone levels, and impaired sperm production, resulting in infertility.

- Y Chromosome Microdeletions

Microdeletions in specific regions of the Y chromosome, particularly the AZF (Azoospermia Factor) region, can cause severe oligospermia or azoospermia, leading to infertility. These microdeletions account for approximately 16% of infertility cases in men with azoospermia or severe oligospermia.

- Cystic Fibrosis Transmembrane Conductance Regulator (CFTR) Gene Mutations

Mutations in the CFTR gene can cause cystic fibrosis, a genetic disorder that primarily affects the lungs and digestive system. In men, CFTR gene mutations can also lead to congenital bilateral absence of the vas deferens (CBAVD), a common cause of male infertility

CHAPTER 3: LIFESTYLE FACTORS

Lifestyle factors play a significant role in determining fertility for both men and women. Several key lifestyle choices can have a profound impact on reproductive health and the ability to conceive.

Lifestyle Factors Affecting Male Fertility

- Smoking

Smoking is one of the most detrimental lifestyle factors for male fertility. Studies have shown that smoking can reduce sperm count, motility, and cause DNA fragmentation within the sperm. The chemicals in cigarette smoke can also impair the function of the tiny hair-like structures (cilia) that help transport sperm. Quitting smoking has been shown to improve sperm quality over time.

- Alcohol Consumption

Excessive alcohol intake has been linked to lower testosterone levels, reduced sperm production, and poorer sperm motility and morphology in men. Even moderate alcohol consumption of just 5 units per week has been associated with adverse effects on sperm quality. Cutting back or eliminating alcohol can help improve male fertility.

- Recreational Drug Use

The use of recreational drugs like marijuana, cocaine, and anabolic steroids can significantly impact male fertility. These substances can disrupt hormone levels, impair sperm production, and lead to DNA damage in sperm. Avoiding recreational drug use is crucial for maintaining male reproductive health.

- Obesity and Weight

Carrying excess weight, as indicated by a high body mass index (BMI), has been associated with reduced sperm count, motility, and morphology in men. Obesity can also contribute to hormonal imbalances that further impair fertility. Achieving and maintaining a healthy weight through diet and exercise can help improve male fertility.

- Stress and Mental Health

Chronic stress and poor mental health can negatively impact male fertility by disrupting the hypothalamic-pituitary-gonadal axis and altering hormone levels. Techniques to manage stress, such as meditation, yoga, and counseling, may help support male reproductive function.

Lifestyle Factors Affecting Female Fertility

- Weight and Nutrition

Both underweight and overweight/obese women can experience fertility challenges. Excess weight is associated with hormonal imbalances, ovulatory dysfunction, and increased risk of conditions like polycystic ovarian syndrome (PCOS). Maintaining a healthy BMI through a balanced diet and regular exercise can optimize female fertility.

- Smoking

Similar to men, smoking can have detrimental effects on female fertility. Smoking has been linked to an increased risk of infertility, earlier menopause, and reduced success rates with assisted reproductive technologies like IVF.

- Alcohol Consumption

Excessive alcohol intake has been shown to disrupt the menstrual cycle, ovulation, and implantation, leading to reduced fertility in women. Limiting or avoiding alcohol is recommended when trying to conceive.

- Stress and Mental Health

High levels of stress can interfere with the delicate hormonal balance required for normal reproductive function in women. Chronic stress can disrupt ovulation, menstrual cycles, and implantation, ultimately impairing fertility. Practicing stress management techniques is important for women trying to conceive.

Lifestyle factors play a crucial role in determining fertility for both men and women. Adopting healthy habits, such as maintaining a healthy weight, avoiding smoking and excessive alcohol, managing stress, and seeking treatment for any underlying medical conditions, can significantly improve the chances of conceiving. Understanding the impact of these lifestyle factors is essential for couples trying to start a family.

CHAPTER 4: AGE RELATED INFERTILITY

Fertility naturally declines with age for both men and women, but the impact of age on reproductive potential is more pronounced in women compared to men.

Age-Related Infertility in Women
A woman's fertility begins to gradually decline around the age of 32, with a more rapid decline starting around age 37. This is primarily due to the natural depletion of a woman's ovarian reserve - the finite number of eggs a woman is born with.

As a woman ages, the quality and quantity of her eggs diminish. Older eggs are more likely to have chromosomal abnormalities, which can lead to increased rates of miscarriage and genetic disorders in offspring. Additionally, the ovaries become less responsive to the hormonal signals that regulate the menstrual cycle and ovulation.

Some key facts about age-related infertility in women:

- By age 30, a woman has lost about 90% of her ovarian reserve compared to when she was born.

- Fertility rates drop significantly after age 35, with a 50% decline in fertility by age 40.
- The chance of conceiving naturally each month drops from around 20% in a woman's 20s to only 5% by age 40.
- The risk of miscarriage increases from around 10-15% in a woman's 20s to 50% by age 45.
- The risk of chromosomal abnormalities like Down syndrome also increases dramatically with maternal age.

Women who delay childbearing until their late 30s or 40s may require the use of assisted reproductive technologies like in vitro fertilization (IVF) to achieve pregnancy. Even with IVF, success rates decline with advancing maternal age.

Age-Related Infertility in Men

While men do not experience the same dramatic decline in fertility with age as women, there are still significant age-related changes that can impact male reproductive potential.

Starting around age 40, men begin to experience a gradual decline in sperm quality and quantity. Some key changes include:

- Decreased sperm motility (ability to swim)

- Increased sperm DNA fragmentation
- Reduced semen volume
- Higher rates of sperm aneuploidy (abnormal chromosome number)

These age-related changes in sperm quality can contribute to decreased fertility, higher rates of miscarriage, and increased risk of genetic disorders in offspring.

However, the impact of male age on fertility is generally less pronounced compared to women. Men can continue to father children well into their 50s and 60s, though the chances of success may decline over time.

Factors Influencing Age-Related Infertility
In addition to the biological changes that occur with aging, other factors can exacerbate age-related infertility in both men and women:

1. Lifestyle factors: Smoking, obesity, excessive alcohol use, and lack of exercise can accelerate the age-related decline in fertility.

2. Medical conditions: Conditions like diabetes, cancer, and sexually transmitted infections can also impair fertility and be more common with advancing age.

3. Environmental exposures: Exposure to toxins, pollutants, and radiation can damage reproductive cells and increase infertility risk.

4. Socioeconomic status: Disparities in access to fertility care and education about age-related infertility can disproportionately impact certain populations.

Strategies to Address Age-Related Infertility
Given the significant impact of age on fertility, several strategies can be employed to help individuals and couples overcome age-related infertility:

1. Education and awareness: Improving public understanding of the effects of age on fertility can encourage earlier family planning and timely access to fertility care.

2. Fertility preservation: Options like egg/sperm/embryo freezing allow individuals to preserve their fertility potential for future use, especially for those who wish to delay childbearing.

3. Assisted reproductive technologies: Techniques like IVF, intrauterine insemination, and

preimplantation genetic testing can help overcome age-related fertility challenges.

4. Lifestyle modifications: Adopting healthy habits like maintaining a healthy weight, quitting smoking, and reducing stress can help optimize fertility at any age.

5. Access to care: Ensuring equitable access to fertility services, including for marginalized populations, is crucial for addressing age-related infertility.

Age-related infertility is a significant public health concern, particularly for women. Understanding the impact of age on fertility, and implementing strategies to address it, is essential for helping individuals and couples achieve their reproductive goals. A multifaceted approach involving education, fertility preservation, assisted reproductive technologies, and lifestyle modifications can help mitigate the effects of age-related infertility.

CHAPTER 5: ENVIRONMENTAL TOXINS

Environmental toxins are a significant contributor to declining fertility rates in both men and women. These toxins, often referred to as endocrine-disrupting chemicals (EDCs), can interfere with the body's hormonal balance and impair reproductive function.

Common Environmental Toxins Affecting Fertility

- Bisphenol A (BPA)

BPA is a chemical found in many plastic products, including food containers, water bottles, and paper receipts. Exposure to BPA has been linked to decreased sperm quality and motility, menstrual cycle disruptions, and increased risk of miscarriage in women.

- Phthalates

Phthalates are chemicals used in the production of plastics, personal care products, and fragrances. Research suggests that phthalate exposure may be associated with decreased sperm quality, impaired ovarian function, and increased risk of infertility.

- Pesticides

Pesticides containing toxic chemicals are widely used in agriculture to control pests and increase crop yield.

Pesticide exposure has been linked to reduced fertility, increased risk of miscarriage, and hormonal disruptions in both men and women.

- Air Pollution

Air pollution in the form of fine particulate matter and toxic gases released from vehicle emissions, industrial processes, and burning fossil fuels can lead to decreased sperm quality, disrupted menstrual cycles, and increased risk of infertility.

- Heavy Metals

Heavy metals such as lead, mercury, and cadmium can accumulate in the body over time and negatively impact reproductive health. Lead exposure, for example, has been associated with reduced fertility in both men and women.

- Flame Retardants

Chemicals found in common flame retardants are used to make clothing or upholstery fire-resistant and may also be found in electronics, nail polish, yoga mats, and other products. Exposure to these chemicals has been linked to altered hormone levels and impaired fertility.

Mechanisms of Action

Environmental toxins can affect fertility through various mechanisms, including:

1. Disrupting the hypothalamic pituitary gonadal (HPG) axis, which regulates hormone production and reproductive function.
2. Exerting estrogenic or anti-androgenic effects, leading to hormonal imbalances.
3. Causing sperm DNA damage and epigenetic changes.
4. Inducing oxidative stress and inflammation, which can impair gamete quality and function.

Impact on Male Fertility

Multiple studies have confirmed a global decline in sperm counts and semen quality in men over the last several decades. This decline cannot be solely attributed to lifestyle factors such as obesity, smoking, and alcohol abuse, but may be partly due to chronic environmental toxin exposures.

Exposure to environmental toxins has been associated with reduced sperm concentration, motility, and morphology[4]. These effects can lead to male infertility and reduced chances of natural conception.

Impact on Female Fertility

Environmental toxins can also negatively impact female fertility. Exposure to EDCs has been linked to menstrual cycle irregularities, ovulatory dysfunction, and increased risk of miscarriage.

Toxins like BPA and phthalates can interfere with ovarian function and disrupt the delicate hormonal balance required for successful conception and pregnancy. Air pollution and heavy metals have also been associated with reduced fertility in women.

Addressing Environmental Toxin Exposure
Reducing exposure to environmental toxins is crucial for preserving fertility in both men and women. Some strategies include:

1. Choosing BPA-free and phthalate-free products whenever possible
2. Opting for organic produce and minimizing pesticide exposure.
3. Using air purifiers and limiting outdoor activities during high pollution days.
4. Avoiding exposure to heavy metals by choosing low-mercury fish, using lead-free cosmetics, and ensuring safe drinking water.
5. Supporting policies and regulations that limit the use of harmful chemicals in consumer products and the environment.

Environmental toxins are a significant threat to male and female fertility. Chronic exposure to EDCs can disrupt hormonal balance, impair gamete quality, and lead to reduced fertility and increased risk of miscarriage. Adopting a proactive approach to reducing toxin exposure, through both individual and societal measures, is crucial for preserving reproductive health and addressing the global decline in fertility rates.

CONCLUSION

Infertility is a complex and multifaceted issue that affects both men and women. While the causes and treatments may differ, it is essential to address infertility holistically, considering the physical, emotional, and social aspects of this condition.

For men, hormonal imbalances, genetic factors, and lifestyle choices can significantly impact fertility. Conditions like low testosterone, varicocele, and sperm abnormalities can impair sperm production and quality, leading to male factor infertility. Treatments for male infertility may involve medications, surgery, or assisted reproductive technologies like sperm retrieval and in vitro fertilization (IVF).

In women, the primary drivers of infertility are often related to ovulatory dysfunction, fallopian tube blockages, and uterine or cervical abnormalities. Hormonal imbalances, such as those seen in polycystic ovarian syndrome (PCOS), can disrupt the menstrual cycle and ovulation, making it difficult to conceive. Fertility treatments for women may include ovulation-stimulating medications, surgical interventions, and assisted reproductive techniques like IVF and intrauterine insemination (IUI).

Regardless of the underlying cause, infertility can have a profound emotional impact on individuals and couples. The stress, anxiety, and feelings of loss associated with the inability to conceive can take a significant toll on mental health. It is crucial for healthcare providers to offer comprehensive support, including access to counseling and support groups, to help patients cope with the challenges of infertility.

Addressing infertility also requires a broader societal approach. Improving access to fertility education, promoting early screening and diagnosis, and ensuring equitable coverage of fertility treatments can help reduce the burden of infertility. Additionally, addressing environmental factors, such as exposure to endocrine-disrupting chemicals, can play a role in preserving reproductive health.